HESI Exit - Test Taking Strategies

By: JCM-HESI Exit Test Preparation Group

This page is intentionally left blank.

This page is intentionally left blank.

Free Online Email Tutoring Services

All preparation booklets purchased directly from JCM Test Preparation Group includes a free four months email tutoring subscription. Any resale of preparation booklets does not qualify for a free email tutoring subscription.

What is Email Tutoring?

Email Tutoring allows buyers to send questions to tutors via email. Buyers can send any questions regarding the exam processes, strategies, content questions, or practice questions.

JCM Test Preparation Group reserves the right not to answer questions with or without reason(s).

How to use Email Tutoring?

Buyers need to send an email to jcmtestpreparationgroup@gmail.com requesting email tutoring services. Buyers may be required to confirm the email address used to purchase the preparation guide or additional information prior to using email tutoring. Once email tutoring subscription is confirmed, buyers will be provided an email address to send questions to. The four months period will start the day the subscription is confirmed.

Any misuse of email tutoring services will result in termination of services. JCM Test Preparation Group reserves the right to terminate email tutoring subscription at anytime with or without notice.

Comments and Suggestions

All comments and suggestions for improvements for the study guide and email tutoring services can be sent to jcmtestpreparationgroup@gmail.com.

This page is intentionally left blank.

Table of Content

This page is intentionally left blank.

Chapter 1 – About the Exam and the Booklet

About the HESI Exit Exam

The HESI Exit Exam is a test to measure the competency of nursing school graduates. The exam is aligned to national standards published by the National Council of State Boards of Nursing, and the exam is used by every U.S. state and Canada to determine entry into nursing practice.

The exam consists of questions related to the following topics: Management of Care, Safety and Infection Control, Health and Promotion and Maintenance, Psychosocial Integrity, Basic Care and Comfort, Pharmacologic and Parenteral Therapies, Reduction of Risk Potential, and Physiologic Adaptation.

What is included in this study guide booklet?

This study guide booklet only contains test taking strategies for the HESI Exit exam. Over 100 strategies are included to support you in passing the HESI Exit exam. The booklet will cover the following topics:

- Study Strategies
- Test Taking Strategies
- Reducing Anxiety Strategies
- Guessing Strategies
- Strategies To Decide Between Two Answers
- Therapeutic Communication Strategies
- Priority Strategies
- Select All That Applies Strategies
- Delegation Strategies

This page is intentionally left blank.

Chapter 2 – Studying Strategies

With any standardized exam, studying smart and right are the key aspects to ensuring your success on the exam. Studying smart allows you to obtain relevant information in a timely manner, which contributes to your success on the exam. Moreover, studying right and smart reduces frustration and anxiety, which are factors that impact scores. The following are studying tips that are extremely useful in your journey to passing the HESI Exit exam.

Studying Strategy 1 – Study the Right Materials

When studying, using the right materials is a critical aspect to increase chances of passing. Remembering and understanding the right content and exam questions will support students to be successful on the exam. Many students buy 1000s of practice questions and 1000s of flashcards, which have nothing to do with the real exam. The human brain is capable of only remembering so much information, especially under time conditions. The best approach is to use the materials and content on the official test website. Or, go with a test preparation company that only specializes in the HESI Exit exam.

Studying Strategy 2 – Dedicate Studying Time

Devoting enough studying time is critical for retention and overall readiness of the exam. Students are very busy with school, job, and/or family, so finding time to study can be a challenge. Best approach is to set a time of the day to devote only for studying. Studying the same time everyday or every other day will keep your schedule consistent. This will prevent you from deferring studying.

Studying Strategy 3 – Avoid Memorizing Everything

Many students have the mindset to memorize everything to be ready for the exam. No one can memorize everything; that is impossible. We recommend that students memorize what is absolutely critical (common lab values or common medications seen on the exam), but focus more on reviewing as oppose to memorizing. For example, if you read a chapter in a book, then 1-2 weeks later, you want to go back and look at the chapter again. The more you look at the content or practice questions the higher the chances you will recall the information. Memorizing everything can be overwhelming and frustrating, so the recommendation is to read, understand, and review.

Studying Strategy 4 – Effective Way to Use Flashcards

Students have a tendency to just go into making a lot flashcards; however, some thought needs to be put into developing flashcards. When used properly, flashcards can be a very helpful tool in the studying process. The best approach is to make flashcards of information you have difficulty recalling or difficulty understanding. We highly discourage making hundreds or thousands of flashcards as that requires too much effort, but also that approach can be ineffective.

Studying Strategy 5 – Study With a Focused Mind

Passing the exam is a critical aspect in reaching aspirations and dreams, so many students will get frustrated and worried about passing. While studying, the best approach is to be focused and positive. Negative distractions while studying is just as bad as distractions during the exam.

Studying Strategy 6 – Focus on Strengths and Weaknesses

You want to focus on weak areas, but you also want to focus on stronger areas while studying. If you have been consistently weak in certain areas, you want to devote time to studying those weak areas. With HESI Exit requirements being to achieve "above passing" in all categories, you want to also focus on studying stronger areas.

Studying Strategy 7 – Second Guessing

Students tend to second guess themselves on the exam all the time. While studying, keep track of the questions you second guess on. This will allow you to see which answer is correct: the first or the second. This will tell you the approach you need to take when completing the real exam.

Studying Strategy 8 – Ask Friends for Insight

Ask your friends who have taken the exam which resources were helpful. Or, ask your friends about topics that were on the exam, so you can study those topics.

Studying Strategy 9 – Best Studying Approach

You want to avoid signing up for 2-3 programs or using 2-3 study guide books. The best approach is to select one study guide or program and stick to the resource. If you are a recent graduate, you want to find a resource that has content but a lot of practice questions. If you have been out of school for many years, you want to start developing your content, so select a resource that is focused on content development. Once you have developed the content, you want to start doing a lot of practice questions.

General Study Tips

1. Don't study sitting on top of a bed.
2. Keep your phone switched off while studying.
3. Get everything (materials, paper, pencil, etc.) needed prior to studying.
4. If you are studying for long periods, take breaks.
5. Find a quiet place to study with little distractions.

This page is intentionally left blank.

Chapter 3 – Test Taking Strategies

The HESI Exit can be very challenging to complete, so good test taking strategies are critical to increase your chances of getting the questions correct. Remember, test taking strategies are not the magic answer to getting all the questions correct; the strategies are to increase your chances of getting the questions correct. With the pressure of completing the exam under time constraints, you can gain knowledge on test taking strategies to smoothly finish the exam without getting stressed during the middle of the test. Below are test taking strategies that can apply for the HESI Exit exam.

Test Taking Strategy 1 – Focus on the Best Answer

Answer choices that are true are not necessary always correct. When taking the exam, you want to focus on the best answer as oppose to true statements.

Test Taking Strategy 2 – Broadest, Most Comprehensive Answer

When unsure about the answer, you want to look for the answer choice that includes all the other answer choices, which is referred to as the "umbrella effect."

Test Taking Strategy 3 – Keep Audience in Mind

If the question mentions the age, eliminate answer choice(s) that is/are not age appropriate.

Test Taking Strategy 4 – Understand the Question

You need to completely read and understand the question before looking at the answer choices. In fact, after understanding the question, you need to think of the answer without looking at the options. After that, you can look at the options and select the answer. If the answer that you thought of was one of the options, that is the one to select.

Test Taking Strategy 5 – Read All Options

Don't rush to select the answer. Completely read and understand each option before making a final decision on the correct answer.

Test Taking Strategy 6 – Negative Words

Play close attention to negative words (ex. not, never, except, least, cannot, won't don't, no, contraindicated, or avoid) or negative phrases (all the following except) in the stem of the question. In this type of question, a correct answer may reflect something that is false.

Test Taking Strategy 7 – Avoid Thinking About Previous Exam Attempts

If you are a repeat test taker, when taking the exam, do not think about your previous attempts. Do not think about what you put as answers in the previous attempts. If you do, your mind will start playing tricks on you, which will impact your score negatively.

Test Taking Strategy 8 – Use Time Wisely

Don't spend too much time on one question. You should attempt to maintain a pace that will allow you to devote enough time to each question. If you find yourself rereading or having difficulty with a given question, select an answer and move forward. Spending too much time on one question may cost you the opportunity to answer other questions that you can actually get correct.

Test Taking Strategy 9 – Good First Impression

The HESI Exit exam requires you to show above passing in all areas of the exam. So, when taking the test, the first ~40 questions are very important. The computer will determine your competency level in certain areas of the exam. If you are not doing well in certain areas, as you continue with the test, the questions will focus more on those struggling areas. Absolutely important, in the beginning, is to read the questions carefully and have a reason why you picked the answers. This will increases chances of getting the questions correct.

Test Taking Strategy 10 – Focus on the Client

You want to remember that as a nurse the reason for undertaking any action with a client is for the best interest of the client. Your primary responsibility is not to preserve the good reputation of the doctor, hospital, nurse, or administrator. If you are having significant difficulty understanding the question or have zero clue what the question is asking, select the option that best supports the client. If you are down to two answer choices, think about which option focuses on the client's needs. If both options focus on the client's needs, look the option that is more positive. Lastly, don't select any answer choice that is dismissive of the client; select an answer that focuses on the client as a worthy human being.

Test Taking Strategy 11 – Focus on Timing of Event

Many students look at common keywords like most, best, least, or first, but they don't look at keywords related to time. You want to pay attention if the question indicates when the event is taking place (preoperative or postoperative; before, during, or after; early or late; prenatal or postpartum). Knowing when the event is taking place can help you to eliminate answer choices or help you select the correct answer.

Test Taking Strategy 12 – Unknown Words

If you encounter a word you do not know in the question, do not panic. Also, don't quickly jump to the conclusion that you will get the question wrong. Read and understand the overall question.

Test Taking Strategy 13 – Avoid Looking At Patterns

Do not look for a pattern in the answers. If you have already selected option A for several questions in a row, do not be reluctant to choose option A again, if you think that it is the correct answer.

Test Taking Strategy 14 – Look for Synonyms

Most likely, exam writers will not use a word from the question in the correct answer choice; that is too easy. However, exam writers might use a synonym in the answer choice that is linked back to a word in the question. The key is to pay attention to synonyms.

Test Taking Strategy 15 – Use the Computer Mouse

To keep yourself focused and prevent yourself from misreading the question, on the computer, you may want to move the mouse under the words as you read.

Test Taking Strategy 16 – Look for Similarities and Groupings

You can look for similarities and groupings in answer choices and the one-of-a-kind key idea in multiple-choice responses. For example, if all the options are related to outdoor activity except for one option, which is related to indoor, then perhaps the correct answer can be the one related to indoor.

Test Taking Strategy 17 – First Action/Priority Questions

When questions have the word first, initial, main, greatest, most, or primary, you have to be careful as more than one answer choice might be true. In such questions, selecting the response with the highest priority is important.

Test Taking Strategy 18 – False Statements

If any part of the answer choice is false, then, the entire statement is false.

Test Taking Strategy 19 – Keep It Simple

Sometimes the obvious answers are overlooked, so keep it simple by not overlooking the obvious answers or reading too much into questions and answer choices. Look for the acceptable, safe, common, and typical response.

Test Taking Strategy 20 – Use True and False Approach

If you are unsure on how to eliminate answer choices, if possible, turn options into true-or-false responses in order to narrow down options.

Test Taking Strategy 21 – No Options Look Correct

Occasionally, you might encounter a question where none of the answer choices look correct. First, you want to determine if the question has a negative or positive tone, and then, find an answer choice that reflects the tone of the question. Or, identify the nursing concept being tested in the question and select the option that closely is related to the nursing concept. Or, select the answer that is linked to the first step of the nursing process, which is related to assessing.

Test Taking Strategy 22 – Similar Answer Choices

Sometimes if two options are extremely similar, neither can be the answer.

Test Taking Strategy 23 –Reasons For Correct and Incorrect Answers

To increase your chances of getting the question correct, make sure that you have a reason as to why the answer is correct. Moreover, have a reason why the other options are incorrect.

Test Taking Strategy 24 – Completely Addresses The Question

Ask yourself whether the option you are considering completely addresses the question. If the option is only partly true or is true only under certain narrow conditions, then it is likely not the right answer.

Test Taking Strategy 25 – Avoid Making Assumptions

If you make an assumption in order for the answer to be true, ask yourself whether this assumption is obvious enough that most test takers will make. If not, don't select that answer.

Test Taking Strategy 26 – Tricky and Deceptive Questions

Some of the test questions can be tricky with two similar right answers. However, the test makers are not purposely writing a question intended to be extremely deceptive. If you suspect that a question is a trick item, make sure you are not reading too much into the question.

Test Taking Strategy 27 – Familiar and Difficult Words

Don't select an answer just because it is the only one with the words you recognize. Exam writers do not put fake words on the test. If you only recognize the words in one option, make sure it is correct and really addresses the question before you choose it. Also, you want to make an effort to dissect difficult words; notice prefixes and suffixes for clues.

Test Taking Strategy 28 – Careful With 100% Qualifiers

On the exam, some answer choices might include 100% qualifiers, such as always, all, everyone, none, never, every, or must. These words imply that there are no exceptions. There are very few instances in which a correct answer is that absolute, so caution has to be taken when these words are included in the answer choices. If you select an answer choice that has a 100% qualifier, you need to be 100% sure that answer is correct. In addition, you also need to have reason why the other options are incorrect.

Test Taking Strategy 29 – Qualifiers That Fall Between Extremes

Some answer choices might include qualifiers that fall between extremes. Some examples include seldom, sometimes, often, frequently, most, many, few, some, usually, generally, and ordinarily. These answer choices are usually true. Moreover, if you narrowed the choices down to two options and one of the options has one of these qualifiers, that option is likely the one to select.

Test Taking Strategy 30 – Legal/Ethical Questions

On the HESI Exit exam, you will encounter questions related to the legal and ethical aspect of nursing. Every situation given on the exam will be different. However, if you are struggling to select an answer, keep the following key aspects in mind:

- Your first priority is always to the client; not to the provider or the institution.
- You want to document everything.
- When you take actions, you want to keep confidentiality in mind.
- As a nurse, you are accountable for all your actions. You should be ready to defend your actions.

When you encounter a legal or ethical question you are struggling with, you want to pick the answer that is most conservative. That is the one answer that benefits the client, but also does not put you in a compromising position.

Test Taking Strategy 31 – Mathematical Questions

HESI Exit is not trying to test your math skills, so if you find yourself spending too much time on the calculation, you are likely doing something wrong. Go back and see if your approach and method to solving is correct. Pay attention to units as some questions might require you to convert to one unit of measurement before performing the calculation to reach the answer. Also, if you are struggling with HESI Exit questions that require math and have to guess, avoid selecting an option that has an extremely high value or an extremely low value.

Test Taking Strategy 32 – Medication Questions

When you see a question on the HESI Exit related to medication administration, keep in mind the 5 rights of medication use: the right patient, the right drug, the right time, the right dose, and the right route.

Test Taking Strategy 33 – Maximize Client Actions

You don't want to always directly do things for the client. A good practice is to engage the client and maximize client's actions. Pay attention to answer choices that have words such as reinforce, support, assist, help, aid, and foster.

Test Taking Strategy 34 – Action Questions

When the question asks for the best action to undertake, that does not automatically indicate to select an answer choice that is an "implementation" type of answer. The answer to the question can be an "assessment" option. Best action to take can be to perform some type of assessment for the client.

Test Taking Strategy 35 – Questions Based on Textbook Practices

Some individuals will have many years of clinical experience or few years of clinical experience. HESI Exit exam is based on textbook practices as oppose to the real world. For example, in the real world, staff, equipment, and resources can be limited, but for the HESI Exit exam, the nurse always has staff, equipment, supplies, and resources. When selecting answers, you want to think about the studying that you did and not your experience working. This is really important when dealing with situational questions on the HESI Exit exam.

Test Taking Strategy 36 – Age Specific Questions

When taking the HESI Exit exam, you want to consider the client to be an adult unless otherwise indicated. If the age of a client is important, the question will include the age.

Test Taking Strategy 37 – Think About Safety

When you encounter questions with more than one answer that could be right, you want to think about safety. Select the answer choice that ensure safety; safety is a priority.

Test Taking Strategy 38 – Types of Questions

On the exam, when dealing with multiple choice questions with only one correct answer, you can categorize those questions in three categories:

1. questions you know the correct answer for nearly 100% certainty
2. questions you think you know but debating between 2 answers
3. questions you absolutely do not know at all

When taking the exam, you don't want to spend too much time on the third type of questions. If you see a question you absolutely do not know, simply guess and move forward. Chances of getting the third type of questions correct are low, so you do not want to waste time on those questions. Plus, your anxiety can increase if you spend too much time on the third type of questions. Focus on questions that you are more likely going to get correct.

This page is intentionally left blank.

Chapter 4 - Reducing Anxiety Strategies

Anxiety is the apprehension over an upcoming event. Anxiety can increase heart rate, cause lack of sleep, and/or poor concentration levels. Test anxiety increases with increased importance, increased likelihood of failing, test proximity, and feeling more unprepared. Having anxiety has played a significant part in many individuals retaking the exam multiple times. Reducing anxiety is a great factor in having a focused mindset along with completing the test in a timely manner. Below are strategies on reducing and managing anxiety.

Importance of Reducing Anxiety Strategy 1 – Be Prepared

Individuals have anxiety because they are not fully ready for the exam. One of the main aspects of reducing anxiety is to study right; you want to be prepared and be organized in your studying. Also, you want to practice the right questions and the right content. Knowing what is on the exam and learning about the exam are one of the key aspects to reducing your anxiety.

Importance of Reducing Anxiety Strategy 2 – Get a Good Night Sleep

Having a good night sleep is critical to support you in reducing anxiety along with establishing a focused mindset. If possible, several days prior to the exam, you want to get in the habit of getting enough sleep. Most importantly, the night before the exam, you want to have a full rest.

Importance of Reducing Anxiety Strategy 3 – Eating Well

Eating healthy days before the exam is critical to support you on your exam date. Most importantly, you want to have a good meal prior to taking the exam to ensure you have the energy to complete the exam.

Importance of Reducing Anxiety Strategy 4 – Do Unrelated Activities

For those with high level anxiety, the recommendation is to do unrelated activities that are fun and distracting the day before the exam. You want to plan your studying to be completed prior to the exam date, and take one day off to relax. Do something away from your studying materials. Meditating or spending time with friends the day before the exam is excellent to undertake.

Importance of Reducing Anxiety Strategy 5 – Be Positive

Throughout the studying process, you want to have a positive mindset. This will allow you to consume knowledge and retain information. Absolutely important is being positive days before the exam, right before the exam, and during the exam.

Importance of Reducing Anxiety Strategy 6 – Techniques to Reduce Anxiety

To reduce anxiety, practice guided imagery, visualization of passing the test, or breathing techniques. While taking the test, if you have high anxiety, take a short 1-2 minutes break to just relax the brain. Or, take a long, slow breath in through your nose.

Importance of Reducing Anxiety Strategy 7 – Avoid Negative Talks

Do not engage in negative talks with anyone before the test. Don't talk to other individuals about being nervous or not studying properly.

Importance of Reducing Anxiety Strategy 8 – Turn Negative Thinking to Positive Thinking

If you have very high anxiety and start thinking negatively, eliminate negative thoughts of self-talk by replacing them with a positive affirmation, such as "I am super ready", "I can do this", or "I studied a lot, so I am ready."

Importance of Reducing Anxiety Strategy 9 – Don't Worry About Other Test Takers

You do not need to worry about other students who finish the test before you do. If you see someone leaving the room within 1 hour of starting the test, do not panic or think about the student leaving so early.

Importance of Reducing Anxiety Strategy 10 – Sit in Comfortable Area

If possible, you want to sit where you feel the most comfortable. If you have high anxiety, try to avoid setting by the door or window as these can be distracters.

Importance of Reducing Anxiety Strategy 11 – Avoid Panicking

Do not panic if you encounter 3-5 questions in a row that you do not know. The key is to try your best and think positive. If you start panicking, that can impact you on other questions as you complete the test.

Importance of Reducing Anxiety Strategy 12 – Mock Practice Test

You want to take a mock practice test under the same conditions as you will on the exam date. Make sure to time yourself and have no distractions as you take the mock test.

This page is intentionally left blank.

Chapter 5 – Guessing Strategies

When taking multiple choice exams, majority of test takers will have to guess at one point. Naturally, knowing the correct answer is the best approach. However, you can be in a situation where you have to guess. There is no 100% guarantee that the guess will be correct, but there are ways to improve your odds of getting the question correct by knowing some effective guessing strategies.

Guessing Strategy 1 – Maximizing Your Score

Let's say you encounter questions you absolutely do not have any clue as to what the questions are asking. These questions are questions you do not understand at all. For those questions, you will be forced into guessing. The key to maximizing your score is to select the same guess for all questions you absolutely do not know. Using the same letter guess only applies to questions you absolutely do not know and cannot eliminate any answer choices. If you can eliminate an answer choice, then you should not use this approach. By using the same guess each time on questions you absolutely do not know, your chances of getting extra few points increases. Again, this strategy only works if you have zero clue what the question is asking. Lastly, this strategy is for multiple choice questions with one correct answer; this does not apply to select all that apply or priority related questions.

Guessing Strategy 2 – Avoid 100% Qualifiers In Guessing

Don't ever guess an option that has 100% qualifiers, such as always, all, everyone, none, never, every, or must.

Guessing Strategy 3 – Avoid Exaggerated or Complex Answers

When guessing, you want to avoid exaggerated or complex answers as those are generally false.

Guessing Strategy 4 – Strongest Answer

When guessing, select the option that you feel is more closely related to the question being asked. Or, select the answer choice that you can link back to your studying.

Guessing Strategy 5 – General Responses

When guessing, you want to avoid selecting general responses as those are typically not the correct answers.

Guessing Strategy 6 – First Instinct

You can always select the answer choice that first caught your eyes.

Guessing Strategy 7 – Two Contradictory Options

When you do not know the best answer and need to guess, look for two contradictory options. One of those options can be the correct answer.

Guessing Strategy 8 – Wording of Question

Just because an option has a word that the question statement includes does not make that option the correct answer. In fact, when guessing, you do not want to pick an answer choice only because it has a word from the question.

Chapter 6 – Strategies To Decide Between Two Answers

The HESI Exit exam does include many questions where there are two options that can be the one correct answer. Many students complain that they don't know how to narrow down to the one correct answer. Others complain that their anxiety increases when they encounter questions with two similar answers. Many of the study guide books or preparation sites do not address how to approach questions with two possible correct answers. Below are some strategies to help determine the correct answer when you have narrowed down to two options. You want to use these strategies in the order presented.

Strategy 1 – Think in Terms of Why One Option is Incorrect

When you have narrowed down to two options, try to think in terms of why one might not be the answer. If you can think of a reason, then that option might not be correct.

Strategy 2 – Contextual Clues

You want to understand the context of the question. More than one answer may look correct, but one will fit the context better.

Strategy 3 – Look at Qualifiers

If you narrowed the choices down to two options and one of the options has one of the qualifiers that fall between extreme qualifiers, that option is likely the one to select.

Strategy 4 – Think About Client's Best Interest

When the question is about a client, you want to pick the answer choice that will impact the client in a more positive manner or support the client in a greater manner.

Strategy 5 – First Action To Take

If you are down to two answer choices, think of which option needs to be taken first regardless if the question asks for the first action.

Strategy 6 - Use Umbrella Effect

When you are down to two answer choices, think about the umbrella effect. See if one option can be completed within the other option.

Strategy 7 - Vividly Imagining

If you are unable to choose between two answers, try vividly imagining the two answer choices. Form a mental image or visualize and sound out the answers. If you are like most people, you will often feel that one of the answers is right. Trust your feeling.

Chapter 7 – Therapeutic Communication Strategies

On the HESI Exit exam, you will encounter questions related to communication between the nurse and the client as that communication relationship is a critical component to treatment. In particular, the exam will have questions related to therapeutic communication, which is described as the face-to-face process of interacting that focuses on improving the physical and emotional well-being of a patient. Therapeutic communication techniques are used by the nurse to provide support and information to patients. Below are some strategies to keep in mind when answering questions related to therapeutic communication on the HESI Exit exam.

Therapeutic Communication Strategy 1 – Don't Make Assumptions

You do not want to assume that the client is purposely being manipulative or is in control of how he or she is feeling. Mental health problems and psychosocial problems can play a factor in the client's behavior whether the client is aware of it or not.

Therapeutic Communication Strategy 2 – Focus on the Client's Concerns

When looking for the correct answer, you want to select an option that directly addresses the concerns of the client. Do not focus on the concerns of the nurse, clinic, or doctor. If the central focus of the question is the client or client's family, the answer you select has to directly address the client or client's family concerns. You also do not want to select an answer choice that takes the focus from the client and puts it on someone else.

Therapeutic Communication Strategy 3 – Seek More Information

You want to look for options that allow open-ended responses and encourage the client to discuss how he or she is feeling. If the client is stressed or has high anxiety, he or she will not be able to immediately state his or her needs or feelings. Having a discussion will give the client opportunity to provide additional information along with give the nurse opportunity to show he or she cares. Also, avoid selecting options that involve closed-ended statements where the client can answer the question in one or two words.

Therapeutic Communication Strategy 4 – Always Validate the Client

You do not want to select any answer choice that dismisses the client in any way. Options that include telling the client "don't worry," "you will be fine," or "the physician knows best" are wrong answers. You also want to avoid selecting options that indicate a short, careless phrase.

Therapeutic Communication Strategy 5 – Be Honest

You do not want to select any answer choice that is dishonest or misleading. You never want to be misleading in any way as that can compromise the nurse-client relationship. You also do not want to select a response that uses coercion to achieve a desired response. For example, don't bribe a child to take his or her medicine with a promise of an chocolate bar.

Therapeutic Communication Strategy 6 – Listen Carefully

A key component of therapeutic communication is listening. Regardless of the client's views, you want to respect the client's beliefs. Responses that tell clients what they should or should not think or do are often incorrect. Keep your views and opinions outside of the conversation with the client.

Therapeutic Communication Strategy 7 – Don't Give Orders

You want to avoid answer choices that directly tell the client what to do. You do not want to select answer choices that push the client to follow advice given.

Therapeutic Communication Strategy 8 – Align with the Client

Look for options that reflect, reinforce, restates, or paraphrase the client's feelings. Also, look for options that encourage the client to describe how he or she is feeling.

Therapeutic Communication Strategy 9 – Avoid Aggressive Communication

Using aggressive language is never therapeutic, but some basic questions starting with "why" or "what were you thinking" can come across as aggressive to the client. Taking this line of questioning presents a verbal presumption that the client has done something wrong; this will discourage the client from expressing his or her feelings.

Therapeutic Communication Strategy 10 – Between Two Answers

When you encounter a therapeutic communication question and you are between two answer choices, you want to select the option with a more positive tone.

This page is intentionally left blank.

Chapter 8 – Priority Strategies

The HESI Exit exam has many priority questions, which test students' ability to identify the highest priority action for the nurse to undertake. For priority questions, multiple answer choices might seem correct; however, you want to select the option that needs to be immediately undertaken to ensure the safe care for the client in the situation presented. Majority, if not all, preparation guides discuss Maslow's hierarchy of needs, the nursing process, and client safety, which this chapter will briefly discuss. In addition, this chapter will provide additional strategies to answer priority questions.

Priority Strategy 1 – Maslow's Hierarchy of Needs

Maslow identifies five levels of human needs, which include physiological, safety or security, love and belonging, esteem, and self-actualization.

- Physiological - these are biological requirements for human survival, such as air, water, food, rest, and health
- Safety and Security – these can be both physical and psychosocial needs; physical needs must come before psychosocial needs
- Love and Belonging – be loved by others and feel accepted by others
- Self-esteem – this is esteem for oneself and respect from others
- Self-actualization – realize personal potential and seek personal growth

The best way to apply Maslow's Hierarchy of Needs to HESI Exit question is to first recognize if answer choices are both physiological and psychosocial. If so, eliminate all psychosocial options. Then, review the remaining options left and eliminate any option that does not relate to the question. Lastly, apply the ABC (airway, breathing, and circulation) technique. If there is an answer choice that addresses airway, then select that option. If not, check to see if there is an answer choice that addresses breathing. If not, check to see if there is an answer choice that addresses cardiovascular system. If the ABC technique does not get you an answer, you want to use process of elimination.

Priority Strategy 2 – The Nursing Process

The first step in the nursing process is assessment. Then, the next process is implementation, which is the care provided to clients. If assessment data is not provided in the question, then you want to select an option that involves assessment and related to the question. If assessment data is provided, then it might be best to look at Maslow's Hierarchy of Needs when selecting the best nursing action.

Priority Strategy 3 – The Safety Aspect

Client safety is a critical aspect for all nurses. This includes safety at hospitals, clinics, home, work, and community. Safety includes meeting the basic needs, which include oxygen, food, fluids, etc. In addition, safety includes reducing hazards that cause injury or decreasing the transmission of pathogens.

Priority Strategy 4 – Knowing a Priority Question

When HESI Exit questions ask which action is the best to take and the assessment aspect is completed, that does indicate that the question is a priority question.

Priority Strategy 5 – Greatest Risk

When a HESI Exit question gives scenarios and ask which client the nurse should attend to first, think in terms of who is at a greater risk of dying if action is not taken, but also think about the likelihood of that happening.

Priority Strategy 6 – Think in Terms of Long Term Complications

Sometime HESI Exit questions will include scenarios where no client is in immediate severe condition. So, you want to think in terms of which client needs have to be addressed first to prevent long term complications.

Priority Strategy 7 – Priority Involves Action

When it comes to priority questions, answer choices that involve notifying or seeking more information are typically not the correct response. Typically, the answer choice that is correct involves an action.

Priority Strategy 8 – Preventing Severe Condition

Some priority questions will involve clients that are not necessarily in immediate severe condition, but require you to identify what further teaching is required, what follow ups are needed, or what clients should do in the future. In such cases, you want to select an answer choice that will prevent the person from getting to that severe condition.

Priority Strategy 9 – Ordering Events or Steps

Some HESI Exit priority questions involve ordering events or steps. The question can ask you to order from highest to lowest priority or lowest to highest priority, so you want to read the question carefully. When ordering events, think in terms of what is necessary to ensure the client remains alive; those are the highest priority actions.

Priority Strategy 10 – Fires

Any priority question that involves fires, use the RACE approach, which includes: remove the clients, then sound the alarm, call the fire department, and finally extinguish the fire. The safety of the clients is the first priority.

This page is intentionally left blank.

Chapter 9 – Select All That Apply Strategies

Select All That Apply (SATA) questions, also known as Multiple-Response Items, are considered the most difficult questions on the HESI Exit. With these types of questions, you will get all or no points; no partial credit is given. Multiple approaches exist to tackle SATA questions, and this chapter is devoted to providing strategies to support you in answering SATA questions.

Select All That Apply Strategy 1 – Options Are Independent

SATA questions do not ask you to choose an option that is better or more complete than other options. Each option should be evaluated on its own and not selected based on the validity of the other options.

Select All That Apply Strategy 2 – True-False Approach

An option that is a true statement may not be the answer associated to the question being asked. When using true-false strategy for SATA questions, you want to be sure that the true statement is linked back to the question.

Select All That Apply Strategy 3 – Keyword Identification Approach

Read the question and pick out keywords. Then, translate, into your own words, the gist of what is being asked in the question. Think about the possible answers without looking at the options. Lastly, skim the answer choices; look for responses that correspond to what first came into your mind.

Select All That Apply Strategy 4 – Best Approach

The following is an effective approach to answering SATA questions:

1. Eliminate all false answers.
2. Of the remaining options, select the options that you know are 100% correct and addresses the question being asked.
3. Of the remaining options, think of reasons why the options might not be correct. If you come up with reasons, then that option is not the answer to select.
4. Of the remaining options, think of reasons why the options might be correct. If you come up with reasons, then that option is the answer to select. After that, any remaining options, do not select those.

This page is intentionally left blank.

Chapter 10 – Delegation Strategies

Delegation is an important aspect of nursing, so the exam does include questions about how to delegate to RN (Registered Nurse), LPN (Licensed Practical Nurse), LVN (Licensed Vocational Nurse), UAP (Unlicensed Assistive Personnel), PCA (Patient Care Attendants), or NAP (Nursing Assistive Personnel – same as CNA and NA). UAPs, PCAs, and nursing assistants must be directly supervised in the provision of safe nursing care while LPNs or LVNs, who are under the supervision of a registered nurse, have more independent in providing nursing care. This chapter contains strategies that are helpful in answering delegation questions for the HESI Exit.

Delegation Strategy 1 – Evaluation, Assessment, and Nursing judgment

Do not delegate functions of evaluation, assessment, and nursing judgment to LVN, LPN, CNA, or nursing assistant. Examples include admitting a client from the operating room to the unit, establishing a plan of care, or handling invasive lines. Functions of evaluation, assessment, and nursing judgment are reserved for RNs to undertake.

Delegation Strategy 2 – Stable and Predictable Outcomes

Activities that can be delegated to LVN, LPN, CNA, or a nursing assistant are those clients who are stable with predictable outcomes. In addition, tasks that involve specific guidelines that are unchanging. Examples include taking vital signs after ambulation, simple dressing changes, or cleaning catheterizations.

Delegation Strategy 3 – Don't Pass the Buck

Make sure that you are not quick to push the tasks to someone else. Think in terms of what nursing action that a nurse can do before calling the doctor.

Delegation Strategy 4 - Five Rights

Start delegation questions with the "Five Right" strategy. To determine if a task may be delegated, consider the following:

1. Is this the **right** task to delegate?
2. Is this the **right** circumstance to delegate?
3. Is this the **right** person to delegate?
4. Is this the **right** direction and communication to ensure successful delegation?
5. Is this the **right** supervision and evaluation associated with the task?

Delegation Strategy 5 - Client Teaching

Any action that requires client teaching must be performed by the RN and cannot be delegated to anyone except another RN.

Delegation Strategy 6 - Begins and Ends with RN

When reading the exam question, always keep in mind that everything begins and ends with the RN.

Delegation Strategy 7 - RN Responsibilities

Keywords like evaluate, assess, determine, teach, instruct, and decide are all things that only the RN can undertake.

Delegation Strategy 8 - Focus on the Client

When answering questions, do not think about what is happening in the rest of the unit or hospital unless it is part of the actual question. The only client to consider in the question is the one involved in that question.

Delegation Strategy 9 - Priority Client

To determine delegation, think in terms of priority client. The priority client is the one individual who is most likely to experience problems or ill effects if not taken care of immediately. You do not want to delegate those clients.

HESI Exit - Test Taking Strategies

CPSIA information can be obtained
at www.ICGtesting.com
Printed in the USA
BVHW041015210620
581999BV00014B/443